This book was compiled by Daniel Melehi
with the A.I assistance of Inventabot

<u>Dedication</u>

I hope this helps all of my wonderful
readers achieve all their goals in their
business. And I would like to thank my
wonderful wife for all of her continued
support in all my ventures.

©Daniel Melehi

May 7 2023

Contents

Chapter 1: The Ego and Its Limitations The concept of the ego has been around for centuries, although it has been interpreted and defined in many different ways. In this chapter, we will explore the ego and its limitations. **Understanding the Ego** The ego is the part of the self that is responsible for our sense of identity and individuality. It shapes our perceptions, thoughts, and behaviors, and helps us navigate the world around us. However, the ego is also limited in its perspective. It tends to see things in terms of duality, such as good vs. bad, right vs. wrong, and us vs. them. This can lead to a narrow and biased view of reality. **The Illusion of the Self** One of the limitations of the ego is that it creates the illusion of a separate self. We often feel like we are separate from others and the world around us. This can lead to feelings of isolation, loneliness, and disconnection. However, upon closer examination, we can see that this sense of separation is illusory. We are interconnected with everything and everyone around us. **The Ego vs. the Soul** While the ego focuses on the individual self, the soul represents a broader perspective that recognizes our interconnectedness with all of existence. The soul is not limited by the duality of the ego and sees the world from a place of unity and love. By transcending the limitations of the ego and connecting with our soul, we can find a deeper sense of meaning and purpose in life. Overall, the ego serves an important role in shaping our individual experiences, but it is limited in its perspective. By recognizing the limitations of the ego and connecting with our soul, we can expand our understanding of reality and find a deeper sense of connection and purpose.

Chapter 1: The Ego and Its Limitations

The ego is a concept that has been central to the understanding of human psychology for many years. In this chapter, we will explore what the ego is, its limitations, and how it affects our lives.

SUBCHAPTER 1.1: UNDERSTANDING THE EGO

The ego is a term used to describe the sense of self that we identify with. It is often described as the "I" or "me" that we experience in our daily lives. The ego is responsible for creating a sense of individuality and separateness from others, which can be both beneficial and limiting. The ego is formed over time, beginning in childhood as a result of our experiences and interactions with the world around us. It is shaped by our family, culture, and society, as well as our own personal choices and experiences.

The Function of the Ego

The ego serves an important function in our lives. It allows us to navigate the world around us, make decisions, and form relationships with others. Without an ego, we would not have a sense of self to distinguish us from others, and we would struggle to interact with the world around us. However, the ego also has its limitations.

SUBCHAPTER 1.2: THE ILLUSION OF THE SELF

One of the limitations of the ego is the illusion of the self. While the ego creates a sense of individuality and separateness from others, it is actually an illusion. The truth is that we are all interconnected and part of a larger whole. Many spiritual traditions have recognized this truth and have developed practices to move beyond the limitations of the ego and experience a sense of unity with the world around us.

Breaking Down the Illusion

Breaking down the illusion of the self can be a difficult process. It requires us to let go of our attachments to our sense of individuality and embrace the larger interconnectedness of the world around us. This can be a frightening and unsettling experience, as it can challenge many of our long-held beliefs and assumptions about ourselves and the world around us. However, it can also be a transformative experience, leading to a deeper sense of connection and purpose in our lives.

SUBCHAPTER 1.3: THE EGO VS. THE SOUL

Another limitation of the ego is its focus on material possessions, status, and external validation. This can lead us to neglect our spiritual needs and fail to recognize the importance of connecting with our inner selves. The soul, on the other hand, represents our spiritual essence and connection to the divine. It is a part of us that cannot be defined by material possessions or external validation, but instead represents our true selves and deepest values.

Finding Balance

Finding balance between the ego and the soul is essential for living a fulfilling life. It requires us to recognize the limitations of the ego and prioritize our spiritual needs. This can be achieved through practices such as meditation, prayer, and introspection. By taking the time to connect with our inner selves and explore our spiritual needs, we can create a more balanced and fulfilling life. Space.Understanding the Ego The concept of the ego has been the subject of numerous discussions and debates over the years. It is a widely used term, but what exactly does it mean? In this subchapter, we will explore the concept of the ego and its limitations. At its most basic level, the ego refers to the part of our consciousness that creates a sense of self. It is what makes us feel separate and distinct from others. The ego is responsible for our sense of identity. It is the voice in our head that says, "I am this" or "I am that." The ego is often associated with the things we identify with, such as our possessions, our job, our social status, and even our beliefs about ourselves. It is also responsible for our emotional states. When we feel criticized or threatened, for example, it is the ego that generates feelings of defensiveness and pride. But while the ego provides a sense of identity, it also has its limitations. One of the biggest limitations of the ego is that it tends to be rooted in fear. The ego is often driven by a need to protect ourselves from harm, whether that harm is physical or emotional. This can lead to defensive and reactive behavior. Another limitation of the ego is that it tends to be concerned with the past and the future, rather than the present moment. The ego is often preoccupied with regrets about the past and worries about the future, which can make it difficult to fully experience the present moment. Overall, while the ego is an important aspect of our consciousness, it is important to understand its limitations. By recognizing the ways in which the ego limits us, we can begin to move beyond it and explore a deeper sense of self. In the following subchapters, we will delve deeper into the illusion of the self and the relationship between the ego and the soul.

THE ILLUSION OF THE SELF

The concept of self is one that has been central to human identity for centuries. However, according to the teachings of many spiritual traditions and modern insights in neuroscience and psychology, the "self" as we commonly understand it may be nothing more than an illusion. Many spiritual teachers and texts suggest that the sense of ego, or "I"-ness, that we identify with is not our true self. Instead, it is a construct that arises from our thoughts, emotions, and actions, and that can be dissolved with the right techniques and insights. In other words, the ego is not a fixed, unchanging entity, but rather a collection of mental patterns and habits. In recent years, scientific research has also shed light on the illusory nature of the self. For example, neuroscientists have found that the brain areas associated with self-reference and self-awareness are highly interconnected and constantly exchanging signals, indicating that the self is not a fixed entity but a dynamic process. Other studies have shown that the brain constructs the sense of self by integrating information from multiple sources, such as sensory input, memories, and social cues. So, if the self is an illusion, what is left? From a spiritual perspective, there is a deeper, more fundamental consciousness that underlies all of existence. This consciousness, variously called the soul, pure awareness, or universal consciousness, is not limited by the boundaries of individual identity. It is the source of all creativity, love, and wisdom, and can be accessed through meditation, prayer, and other spiritual practices. Recognizing the illusion of the self can be an important step on the path to spiritual awakening. By letting go of attachment to the ego and realizing our true nature as part of a larger whole, we can experience greater peace, compassion, and joy in our lives.

SUBCHAPTER 1.3: THE EGO VS. THE SOUL

The ego and soul are two opposing forces within us that shape our perception of the world and ourselves. While the ego is the part of us that is focused on our individual needs and desires, the soul represents our higher self and spiritual nature. The ego is concerned with external validation, material possessions, and achieving personal success. It is driven by fear, need for control, and self-importance. The ego often causes us to feel separate from others and creates a sense of competition and comparison. On the other hand, the soul is concerned with our spiritual growth and understanding. It is driven by love, compassion, and connection. The soul recognizes the interconnectedness of all beings and seeks to help and uplift others. When we are stuck in ego consciousness, we become trapped in a cycle of wanting more and feeling unfulfilled. We may also experience negative emotions such as jealousy, anger, and greed. However, when we are in touch with our soul, we experience inner peace, contentment, and gratitude. Psychedelic experiences have been known to help individuals transcend the limitations of the ego and connect with their higher selves. By dissolving barriers and allowing for a deeper connection to the universe, psychedelics offer individuals the opportunity to shed their egos and explore their spiritual nature. Ultimately, the goal is not to eliminate the ego completely but to integrate it with the soul so that our actions align with our inner truth and purpose. Through mindfulness, meditation, and other spiritual practices, we can cultivate a greater sense of awareness and connection to our true selves. In doing so, we can begin to live a life that is more in alignment with our higher purpose and soul's calling.

Chapter 2: Psychedelics and Their Effects

Psychedelics are a class of drugs that are known to elicit profound changes in perception, mood, and thought. They produce their effects primarily by altering the activity of neurotransmitters in the brain such as serotonin, dopamine, and norepinephrine. There are various types of psychedelics that differ in their chemical structure and mechanism of action.

SUBCHAPTER 2.1: BRIEF HISTORY OF PSYCHEDELICS

Psychedelics have been used for thousands of years in various cultures for religious, shamanic, and healing purposes. The use of psychedelics by indigenous cultures dates back to prehistoric times. In the 20th century, a new era of psychedelic use emerged in the Western world with the discovery of LSD by Albert Hofmann in 1938. During the 1950s and 1960s, psychedelics gained popularity in the counterculture movement and were used as a means of exploring altered states of consciousness and as a tool for personal and spiritual growth.

SUBCHAPTER 2.2: TYPES OF PSYCHEDELICS

There are several types of psychedelics that can be classified based on their chemical structure and mechanism of action. Some of the most commonly used psychedelics include:

Lysergic acid diethylamide (LSD)

LSD is a synthetic compound that is chemically similar to serotonin. It is known for its profound and long-lasting effects, which can last up to 12 hours. It is also one of the most potent psychedelics, with doses as low as 20 micrograms capable of producing significant effects.

Magic mushrooms (Psilocybin)

Psilocybin is a naturally occurring compound found in certain species of mushrooms. It is a prodrug that is converted to psilocin in the body, which is responsible for its psychedelic effects. Magic mushrooms are one of the oldest known psychedelics, with use dating back to prehistoric times.

Mescaline

Mescaline is a naturally occurring compound found in the peyote cactus and certain other plants. It has been used by indigenous cultures in Central and North America for centuries for religious and healing purposes.

SUBCHAPTER 2.3: MECHANISMS OF PSYCHEDELICS

Psychedelics primarily act on the serotonin system in the brain, particularly the 5-HT2A receptor subtype. They bind to these receptors and activate them, leading to a cascade of effects that alter the activity of other neurotransmitters such as dopamine and norepinephrine. This leads to changes in perception, mood, thought, and behavior that are characteristic of the psychedelic experience.

SUBCHAPTER 2.4: PSYCHOLOGICAL AND PHYSICAL EFFECTS

Psychedelics can produce a wide range of psychological and physical effects. Some common effects include:

Psychedelic Effects

- Altered perception of time and space
- Visual and auditory hallucinations
- Intense emotions and mood changes
- Alteration of thought processes and language
- Changes in sense of self and ego dissolution

Physical Effects

- Dilated pupils
- Rapid heartbeat
- Increase in blood pressure
- Nausea and vomiting
- Increased body temperature and sweating

It is important to note that the effects of psychedelics can vary widely depending on the dose, setting, and individual factors such as personality, mood, and mindset. In some cases, the effects can be intense and overwhelming, which can lead to negative or adverse experiences. It is therefore important to approach the use of psychedelics with caution and under the guidance of a qualified professional.

SUBCHAPTER 2.1: BRIEF HISTORY OF PSYCHEDELICS

Psychedelics have been used by humans for centuries, if not millennia, for various purposes. One of the earliest recorded uses of psychedelics was by ancient civilizations in Mesoamerica, where psilocybin mushrooms were used ceremonially in religious practices. The indigenous people of the Amazon basin also used ayahuasca, a brew made from the Banisteriopsis caapi vine, for divinatory and healing purposes. In the modern era, the use of psychedelics gained mainstream popularity in the mid-20th century. In 1943, Swiss chemist Albert Hofmann synthesized lysergic acid diethylamide (LSD) while studying ergot alkaloids. Hofmann later accidentally ingested a small amount of LSD and experienced its psychedelic effects, leading to further research and experimentation with the substance. In the 1950s and 1960s, psychedelic substances such as LSD, psilocybin, mescaline, and DMT gained popularity among countercultural movements, particularly in the United States and Europe. The cultural phenomenon of the "Summer of Love" in 1967, centered in San Francisco's Haight-Ashbury neighborhood, was associated with the use of LSD and other psychedelics. However, the increasing use of psychedelics also led to concerns about their safety and potential for abuse. The US government declared LSD a Schedule I controlled substance in 1970, effectively criminalizing its possession and use. Despite this legal crackdown, research into the therapeutic potential of psychedelics continued in various forms. In the 1990s, a team of researchers led by Rick Strassman conducted a groundbreaking study on the effects of DMT, the active ingredient in ayahuasca. More recently, a resurgence of interest in psychedelic research has led to studies on the use of substances such as psilocybin and MDMA for treating conditions such as depression, anxiety, and PTSD. The history of psychedelics is complex and varied, with both positive and negative aspects. The use of these substances has been associated with spiritual and creative experiences, as well as concerns about safety and legal issues. Nonetheless, the continued interest in psychedelics suggests that their potential benefits and risks remain an important area of inquiry.

SUBCHAPTER 2.2: TYPES OF PSYCHEDELICS

There are several types of psychedelics that have been studied for their effects on the human mind. Each of these substances has its unique characteristics and produces different experiences. Here are some of the most notable psychedelics:

LSD (Lysergic acid diethylamide)

LSD is a synthetic substance that was first synthesized in 1938. It is known for its profound psychedelic effects, which can last for up to 12 hours. LSD is typically ingested orally, either as a sheet of blotting paper or a liquid substance. It can cause visual hallucinations, altered perceptions, and profound changes in one's sense of self and reality.

Mushrooms

Mushrooms containing psilocybin have been used for centuries for their psychedelic effects. They are typically ingested orally in their natural form or dried and consumed as a tea. Psilocybin mushrooms have similar effects to LSD, but they tend to be more introspective and emotional. The trip typically lasts between 4 to 6 hours.

DMT (Dimethyltryptamine)

DMT is a powerful psychedelic substance that is naturally occurring in several plants and animals. It can be smoked, injected, or ingested orally in combination with other substances or as a brew. DMT is known for its intense and short-lived effects that usually last about 20 to 30 minutes. People often report spiritual experiences and feelings of transcendence while under its influence.

MDMA (3,4-Methylenedioxymethamphetamine)

MDMA is a synthetic substance that is commonly known as a party drug or ecstasy. It produces feelings of empathy, love, and euphoria. MDMA is typically ingested orally in the form of a tablet or capsule. It is not considered a classical psychedelic, but it has been studied for its therapeutic potential in treating mental health disorders such as PTSD.

Mescaline

Mescaline is a naturally occurring psychedelic substance that is found in several species of cactus. It produces visual and perceptual changes similar to LSD and psilocybin mushrooms. Mescaline is typically ingested orally as a tea or extracted from the cactus and consumed as a powder.

Ayahuasca

Ayahuasca is a powerful psychedelic brew that has been used in shamanic rituals and spiritual practices in South America for centuries. It is made from a combination of plants containing dimethyltryptamine and monoamine oxidase inhibitors or MAOIs. The MAOIs allow the DMT to remain active when ingested orally. Ayahuasca produces a long-lasting, intense, and often transformative experience that can last up to 8 hours. Understanding the different types of psychedelics and their effects is essential in determining the appropriate substance for research or personal use. It is also important to note that these substances can have varying effects based on individual factors such as dosage, mental and physical health, and the setting in which they are consumed.

SUBCHAPTER 2.3:
MECHANISMS OF
PSYCHEDELICS

The mechanisms of psychedelics are still not fully understood by scientists and researchers. However, there are several theories that attempt to explain how these substances work within the brain. One of the most popular theories is that psychedelics affect serotonin, a neurotransmitter found in the brain that is involved in regulating mood, appetite, and sleep. Specifically, psychedelics appear to activate serotonin receptors in the prefrontal cortex, which is responsible for many cognitive functions such as decision-making, attention, and social behavior. This activation of serotonin receptors leads to an increase in activity within the prefrontal cortex, which can result in altered perceptions, emotions, and thoughts. Additionally, psychedelics may also reduce activity in the default mode network

(DMN), a group of interconnected brain regions that become active when a person is at rest and not focused on the outside world. By reducing activity within the DMN, psychedelics may enable greater connectivity and communication between different regions of the brain, leading to novel insights and experiences. Another theory is that psychedelics enhance neuroplasticity, the brain's ability to adapt and change in response to experiences. This may be due to the selective activation and integration of neural pathways that are not normally utilized, leading to greater flexibility and openness of the mind. Overall, the mechanisms of psychedelics are complex and multifaceted, and further research is needed to fully understand how they work within the brain.

SUBCHAPTER 2.4: PSYCHOLOGICAL AND PHYSICAL EFFECTS

Psychedelics have been known to elicit a wide array of psychological and physical effects. These effects can vary greatly depending on the specific type of psychedelic used, the dose, and the setting in which it is taken. In this section, we will explore some of the most common psychological and physical effects associated with the use of psychedelics.

Psychological Effects

One of the most notable psychological effects of psychedelics is an altered state of consciousness. Users often describe this state as a feeling of oneness with the universe or a sense of interconnectedness with all things. They may also experience a heightened sense of creativity, increased empathy and emotional sensitivity, and a more profound understanding of themselves and their place in the world. Another common psychological effect of psychedelics is the experience of hallucinations. These can range from mild visual distortions to vivid, full-blown hallucinations that are indistinguishable from reality. Users may see patterns, colors, and fractals, or they may have more complex visual experiences, such as visions of other worlds or encounters with spiritual beings. While many of these psychological effects can be positive and enlightening, some users may also experience negative psychological effects. These can include feelings of fear, anxiety, paranoia, or even a loss of control. Users who have pre-existing mental health conditions may be at a higher risk of experiencing negative psychological effects while using psychedelics.

Physical Effects

Alongside the psychological effects of psychedelics, there are also various physical effects that users may encounter. These can include changes in heart rate and blood pressure, dilation of the pupils, and changes in body temperature. Some users may also experience nausea, vomiting, or diarrhea, particularly if they have consumed a large dose of a psychedelic. Perhaps the most significant physical effect of psychedelics is the alteration of sensory perception. Users may experience changes in their perception of time, space, and their physical environment. They may also experience synesthesia, a phenomenon where senses become cross-wired, such as seeing music or tasting colors. It's important to note that the physical effects of psychedelics can be unpredictable, and that proper precautions, such as ensuring a safe and comfortable setting, are essential to minimizing potential risks.

Conclusion

Psychedelics can elicit a wide range of psychological and physical effects, both positive and negative. It's important to understand these effects and the potential risks associated with psychedelic use before deciding to partake in them. In the next chapter, we will delve deeper into the role of psychedelics in spiritual practices and their potential for inducing spiritual experiences.

Chapter 3: Psychedelics and Spiritual Awakening

Psychedelics have been used for centuries by various cultures to induce altered states of consciousness, often with the purpose of spiritual and religious experiences. In recent years, research into the therapeutic potential of psychedelics has gained traction, with many studies pointing to the ability of these substances to facilitate profound spiritual awakenings in individuals. This chapter explores the role of psychedelics in spiritual awakening and the scientific basis behind their efficacy.

SUBCHAPTER 3.1: THE ROLE OF PSYCHEDELICS IN SPIRITUAL PRACTICES

Many spiritual traditions involve the use of psychedelics or other mind-altering substances to facilitate heightened states of consciousness. In some cultures, it is believed that these substances are gifts from the gods and that their use can lead to transcendence and spiritual insight. Psychedelics can provide a shortcut to achieving spiritual experiences that may take years of meditation or other practices to attain.

SUBCHAPTER 3.2: SPIRITUAL EXPERIENCES ON PSYCHEDELICS

One of the most profound effects of psychedelics is the ability to induce mystical or spiritual experiences. These experiences are characterized by a sense of interconnectedness with all things, a loss of ego boundaries, and an altered sense of time and space. Many people report feeling a sense of awe and wonder at the beauty and complexity of the universe, as well as a deep sense of peace and love.

SUBCHAPTER 3.3: THE SCIENCE OF PSYCHEDELIC-ASSISTED THERAPY

In recent years, there has been a renewed interest in the therapeutic potential of psychedelics for a range of mental health conditions, including depression, anxiety, and PTSD. Studies have shown that psychedelics can stimulate the growth of new brain cells and enhance brain plasticity, which may explain their ability to promote healing and change in individuals. Psychedelic-assisted therapy involves the use of these substances under controlled conditions, with the guidance of a trained therapist.

SUBCHAPTER 3.4: THE INTEGRATION OF PSYCHEDELIC EXPERIENCES

While psychedelics can induce powerful spiritual experiences, integrating these experiences into everyday life can be a challenge. Many people report that the insights they gain from psychedelics can be difficult to translate into actionable changes in behavior or lifestyle. Integration involves taking the insights gained from psychedelic experiences and applying them to daily life, through practices such as meditation, self-reflection, and community support. Overall, the use of psychedelics in spiritual and therapeutic contexts is a promising area of research that has the potential to revolutionize our understanding of consciousness and the human mind. However, as with any powerful tool, caution is necessary, and the risks and benefits of psychedelic use must be carefully considered.

THE ROLE OF PSYCHEDELICS IN SPIRITUAL PRACTICES

For centuries, spiritual seekers have looked for ways to connect with the divine. Practices such as meditation, prayer, and fasting have been used to achieve altered states of consciousness and gain access to higher realms of spiritual understanding. However, the use of psychedelics, such as LSD, psilocybin, and ayahuasca, has gained increasing attention in recent years as a powerful tool for spiritual exploration. Many people who have used psychedelics report profound mystical experiences that have transformed their understanding of the world. These experiences often involve a sense of unity with all things and a feeling of transcendence beyond the limited individual self. In this way, psychedelic experiences can help individuals break free from the rigid confines of ego and connect with something larger and more meaningful. Some proponents of psychedelics argue that they can provide a shortcut to spiritual awakening, allowing individuals to experience in a matter of hours what might take years of dedicated spiritual practice to achieve. Many people report feeling more connected to nature, more empathetic towards others, and more in touch with their own inner truth after using psychedelics. However, it's important to recognize that psychedelics can be a double-edged sword. While they have the potential to bring about positive spiritual experiences, they can also lead to difficult or even traumatic experiences. As such, it's important to approach these substances with caution and with a deep respect for their power. Additionally, the use of psychedelics in spiritual practice isn't without controversy. Many religions and spiritual traditions have strict guidelines around the use of mind-altering substances, and some argue that using psychedelics for spiritual purposes is a form of "cheating" or a shortcut that ultimately falls short of genuine spiritual progress. Despite these concerns, the use of psychedelics in spiritual exploration continues to gain popularity and recognition. As our understanding of the human mind and consciousness expands, it's clear that these substances have an important role to play in shaping our understanding of spirituality and our place in the world.

SUBCHAPTER 3.2: SPIRITUAL EXPERIENCES ON PSYCHEDELICS

The use of psychedelics has been linked to spiritual experiences by many users. These experiences can be profound and life-changing, often leading to a greater sense of self-awareness and connectedness to the world around us. During a psychedelic experience, users may report feeling a sense of being connected to a higher power or the universe itself. They may also report feeling a sense of oneness with all things, leading to a greater appreciation and deeper understanding of the interconnectedness of all living things. Some users may also report a sense of ego dissolution, which can be enlightening as it allows the user to see beyond the limitations of their individual self and become more open to new perspectives and ideas. Spiritual experiences on psychedelics can also be accompanied by profound emotions such as love, bliss, and a deep sense of peace. These experiences can be incredibly healing for individuals suffering from anxiety, depression, and other mental health conditions. However, it's important to note that not all spiritual experiences on psychedelics are positive. Some users may encounter challenging or difficult experiences, termed "bad trips", which can be scary or overwhelming. It's important for individuals to be prepared for the possibility of a difficult experience and to have a trusted guide or therapist present to help them navigate through it. Overall, spiritual experiences on psychedelics can be a powerful tool for personal growth and self-discovery. However, it's important to approach these experiences with caution and respect for the substances and their potential risks. In the next subchapter, we will explore the science behind psychedelic-assisted therapy and its potential for spiritual healing.

SUBCHAPTER 3.3: THE SCIENCE OF PSYCHEDELIC-ASSISTED THERAPY

Psychedelic-assisted therapy is a relatively new field of study in the medical world that has shown promising results in treating various mental health disorders. The use of psychedelics in therapy was first introduced in the 1950s, but after some negative publicity and a lack of regulation, it was banned in the 1970s. However, recent scientific studies have brought the use of psychedelics in therapy back into the spotlight. Studies have shown that psychedelic-assisted therapy can be effective in treating depression, anxiety, addiction, and PTSD. The use of psychedelics, such as MDMA, psilocybin, and LSD, can help patients to confront and process past traumatic experiences and negative thought patterns. This can lead to significant improvements in psychological functioning and emotional well-being. Researchers believe that psychedelics work by interacting with the default mode network (DMN) in the brain. The DMN is responsible for our sense of self and our perception of the world around us. When someone experiences depression, anxiety, or other mental health issues, the DMN becomes overactive, leading to negative rumination and an inability to see things in a positive light. Psychedelics are believed to inhibit the DMN, allowing for new neural connections to form and paving the way towards more positive thought processes. Psychedelic-assisted therapy is not a one-size-fits-all treatment and should only be administered by a licensed healthcare professional in a controlled environment. Patients must also undergo careful preparation and integration to ensure the best possible outcomes. However, the results show that psychedelic-assisted therapy has the potential to revolutionize the field of mental health treatment and provide hope for those who struggle with debilitating mental health issues.

SUBCHAPTER 3.4: THE INTEGRATION OF PSYCHEDELIC EXPERIENCES

Integrating psychedelic experiences can often be a challenging process, but it can also be one of the most rewarding experiences a person can have. Integrating psychedelic experiences refers to the process of making sense of, and applying, insights and realizations gained during a psychedelic experience into one's daily life. This process typically involves a period of reflection, meditation, and journaling. It is also important to have the support and guidance of a therapist or experienced facilitator during the integration process. One of the key benefits of integrating psychedelic experiences is a lasting transformation on one's view of the world and their place in it. This can lead to a greater sense of purpose, improved relationships, and an increased sense of interconnectedness with all life. However, without proper integration, the insights gained during a psychedelic experience may fade away, leading to a sense of confusion and disorientation. It is important to approach the integration process with an open mind and a willingness to change. This includes making lifestyle changes that support one's newfound insights and values. For example, if one realizes during a psychedelic experience that they have been neglecting important relationships in their life, they may need to make changes to their daily routine or priorities in order to prioritize those relationships going forward. Psychedelic integration can also involve exploring spiritual practices such as meditation, yoga, and prayer. These practices can help deepen one's connection to their inner self and to the world around them. By incorporating these practices into daily life, one can continue to nurture their spiritual growth and development. In summary, the integration of psychedelic experiences is a critical step in the journey towards personal growth and spiritual awakening. It requires a willingness to reflect deeply on one's experiences and a commitment to making lasting lifestyle changes based on the insights gained. With proper guidance and support, psychedelic integration can be a transformative and empowering process.

Chapter 4: The Challenges and Risks of Psychedelic Use

Psychedelics have gained popularity in recent years as a tool for personal growth and spiritual awakening. While they have shown promising results in treating mental health disorders, their use is not without risks. In this chapter, we will explore some of the challenges and risks associated with psychedelic use.

SUBCHAPTER 4.1: LEGAL AND POLITICAL OBSTACLES

One of the biggest obstacles to psychedelic use is their legal status. The majority of psychedelics are classified as Schedule I drugs, which are considered to have a high potential for abuse and no accepted medical use. This classification makes it difficult for researchers to study their therapeutic potential and for individuals to access them for personal use. In recent years, there have been some positive developments in this area. Some jurisdictions have decriminalized or legalized the use of certain psychedelics, and there is a growing movement for reform at the national level. However, there is still a long way to go before psychedelics are widely accepted and accessible.

SUBCHAPTER 4.2: PERSONAL RISKS OF PSYCHEDELIC USE

Psychedelics can be powerful tools for personal growth and healing, but they also come with certain risks. One of the main risks is the potential for a challenging or "bad" trip. This can be caused by a variety of factors, such as an inappropriate setting or dose, preexisting mental health conditions, or a lack of preparation or integration. Other risks include the potential for physical harm, such as falls or accidents while under the influence, as well as the possibility of legal consequences. Additionally, some individuals may experience persistent psychological effects, such as flashbacks or HPPD (Hallucinogen Persisting Perception Disorder).

SUBCHAPTER 4.3: AVOIDING NEGATIVE EXPERIENCES

While there is no guaranteed way to avoid a challenging trip, there are certain steps that can be taken to minimize the risk. One of the most important factors is set and setting. This refers to the mindset and physical environment in which the psychedelic experience takes place. Other factors that can help reduce the risk of a challenging trip include choosing the right dose, having a trusted and experienced trip sitter present, and engaging in proper preparation and integration practices.

SUBCHAPTER 4.4: HARM REDUCTION STRATEGIES

Even with the best preparation, there is still a risk of a challenging trip. In these situations, it is important to have strategies for harm reduction. This can include using grounding techniques, such as deep breathing or meditation, changing the physical environment, or seeking support from a trusted friend or therapist. It is also important to have access to emergency medical care in case of physical harm or a mental health crisis. Having a plan in place and knowing where to seek help can make all the difference in a difficult situation.

Conclusion

While there are certainly risks associated with psychedelic use, they can be minimized through proper preparation and harm reduction strategies. With continued research and advocacy, psychedelics have the potential to play a valuable role in mental health treatment and spiritual growth. It is up to individuals and society as a whole to navigate these challenges and embrace the potential benefits of these powerful substances.Legal and Political Obstacles: One of the biggest challenges facing the use of psychedelics is their legal and political status. Most countries have strict laws in place that prohibit the possession, manufacture, and sale of such substances. These laws are often based on outdated ideas of drug use and addiction, and they fail to take into account the potential benefits that psychedelics can offer. In recent years, there has been a push to legalize and decriminalize the use of psychedelics. Several cities in the United States have already taken steps towards decriminalization, and there are ongoing efforts to remove federal restrictions on medical research involving psychedelics. However, these efforts face significant opposition from politicians and policymakers who view drugs as inherently dangerous and addictive. There is also the concern that legalizing psychedelics could lead to increased recreational use, which could lead to greater risk of harm. Despite these obstacles, advocates for the use of psychedelics continue to make progress in changing the conversation around these substances. They argue that psychedelics can be used safely and responsibly, and that their potential benefits far outweigh any potential risks. In the coming years, it is likely that we will continue to see a shift in attitudes towards psychedelics, both in terms of their legal status and their acceptance as a valid tool for personal and spiritual growth. As more research is conducted and more people share their positive experiences, we may see a future where psychedelics are widely accepted and available for those who wish to explore their inner selves.

SUBCHAPTER 4.2: PERSONAL RISKS OF PSYCHEDELIC USE

While psychedelics have shown promising results in promoting spiritual awakening and personal growth, they also come with personal risks. Like any powerful tool, psychedelics should be used with caution and respect. One of the main personal risks of psychedelic use is the possibility of a "bad trip." A bad trip can occur when a person experiences intense anxiety, paranoia, or other negative emotions while under the influence of a psychedelic. This can be a terrifying and traumatic experience, and can lead to long-term psychological damage if not properly addressed. Another risk of psychedelic use is the potential for physical harm. Certain psychedelics can cause physical symptoms such as nausea, vomiting, and increased heart rate, which can be dangerous for individuals with certain medical conditions. Additionally, the long-term effects of frequent psychedelic use on the body are not yet fully understood. Psychedelics can also have a profound impact on an individual's perception of reality. While this can be a positive experience for many, it also has the potential to lead to delusional thinking or detachment from reality. This can be especially detrimental for individuals with pre-existing mental health conditions such as schizophrenia. It is important to note that psychedelic use is not recommended for everyone. Individuals with a family history of mental illness or other risk factors may be more susceptible to negative side effects. It is crucial for individuals to do their research and consult with a healthcare professional before deciding to use psychedelics. Overall, while psychedelics have the potential to provide profound and life-changing experiences, it is important to approach them with caution and respect. By understanding the personal risks involved and taking proper precautions, individuals can maximize the potential benefits while minimizing the potential harm.

SUBCHAPTER 4.3: AVOIDING NEGATIVE EXPERIENCES

While psychedelic experiences can be transformative and life-changing, they can also be overwhelming and challenging. It's important to take steps to avoid negative experiences and minimize risks when using psychedelics. One of the most important factors in avoiding negative experiences is setting. It's important to create a comfortable, safe environment for the psychedelic experience. This can include things like choosing a comfortable and familiar setting, such as one's own home or a trusted friend's home. It's also important to ensure that the environment is free from any potential stressors, such as loud noises or unexpected visitors. Another important factor is mindset. Ensuring that one is in a positive and relaxed state of mind before the experience can go a long way towards mitigating potential negative experiences. Mindfulness practices, such as meditation or deep breathing exercises, can help to calm the mind and reduce anxiety. In addition to environmental and mental factors, it's important to consider dosage and substance choice when trying to avoid negative experiences. Starting with a low dose and gradually increasing over time can help to mitigate the risk of overwhelming experiences. Additionally, choosing a reputable source for psychedelic substances and doing research on the substance beforehand can help to ensure a more positive experience. Finally, it's important to have a trusted and reliable person present during the experience. This person can serve as a source of support and guidance if needed, and can help to ensure the safety and well-being of the person using psychedelics. By taking these steps to minimize risks and ensure a positive set and setting, it's possible to have transformative and life-changing experiences with psychedelics.

SUBCHAPTER 4.4: HARM REDUCTION STRATEGIES

While psychedelic use can offer many benefits, there are also potential risks involved. As such, it's important to understand and implement harm reduction strategies when using these substances. One of the most effective harm reduction strategies is proper preparation. This involves researching the substance being used, its effects and dosages, and any potential interactions with medications. It's also important to consider the setting and environment in which the psychedelic experience will occur. During the experience, it can be helpful to have a trusted and sober guide present. They can help ensure a safe and comfortable environment and handle any unexpected situations that may arise. Another important harm reduction strategy is ensuring proper dosage. Starting with a lower dose and slowly increasing can help avoid overwhelming experiences. It's also recommended to have a scale to accurately measure dosage and avoid accidentally taking too much. In the event of a challenging or difficult experience, having a plan in place can help minimize harm and ensure a safe return to reality. This may involve having calming music or a comforting object on hand, or having a trusted friend or therapist to call for support. Overall, harm reduction strategies can help ensure a safe and positive experience with psychedelics. Proper preparation, dosage, and support can all contribute to a successful and beneficial experience.

Chapter 5: Beyond the Ego: A New Paradigm

The human ego has been a central focus of spiritual and psychological exploration for centuries. It is the aspect of our psyche that creates a sense of self and gives us a sense of purpose in life. However, many spiritual traditions suggest that the ego can also be a hindrance to our spiritual growth, leading us down a path of self-centeredness and separation from the world around us. Psychedelics can play a powerful role in helping to transcend the ego and move us towards a new paradigm of spiritual awakening.

SUBCHAPTER 5.1: TRANSCENDING THE EGO

Transcending the ego is a concept that can be difficult to grasp, as it involves letting go of our attachment to our individual identity and embracing a larger sense of oneness with the universe. Psychedelic experiences can be a powerful catalyst for this transformation, as they can dissolve the boundaries between self and other, leading to a sense of unity and interconnectedness. This sense of unity can have profound implications for our well-being and relationships with others, allowing us to connect with the world around us in a more meaningful way.

SUBCHAPTER 5.2: LIVING FROM THE SOUL

Living from the soul is another aspect of the new paradigm of spiritual awakening that can be facilitated by psychedelic experiences. The soul can be thought of as our higher self, our true essence that goes beyond the limitations of the ego. When we live from the soul, we act with greater compassion, kindness, and love, and are guided by a deeper sense of purpose. Psychedelics can help us access this state of being, allowing us to tap into our spiritual nature and live more authentic, fulfilling lives.

SUBCHAPTER 5.3: IMPLICATIONS FOR SOCIETY AND CULTURE

The implications of this new paradigm of spiritual awakening are far-reaching, with potential implications for society and culture as a whole. As more people begin to explore the possibilities of transcending the ego and living from the soul, we may see a shift towards a more compassionate, interconnected world. This could have a positive impact on issues such as social justice, environmentalism, and global peace, as people become more attuned to the needs of others and the world around them.

SUBCHAPTER 5.4: THE FUTURE OF PSYCHEDELIC RESEARCH AND ADVOCACY

The future of psychedelic research and advocacy is bright, as more and more people recognize the potential benefits of these substances for spiritual and psychological growth. As research continues to shed light on the mechanisms and effects of psychedelics, we can expect to see more widespread acceptance and use of these substances, both within the spiritual community and beyond. However, it is important to continue advocating for responsible use and harm reduction strategies, as well as working towards legal reform to ensure safe and accessible use of psychedelics for those who wish to explore their potential for spiritual awakening. Overall, the new paradigm of spiritual awakening that is emerging through the use of psychedelics offers a powerful perspective on the possibilities of human growth and evolution. By transcending the ego and living from the soul, we can connect with a deeper sense of purpose, meaning, and interconnection, both within ourselves and the world around us.

SUBCHAPTER 5.1: TRANSCENDING THE EGO

Transcending the ego is one of the core goals of many spiritual traditions. The ego is often viewed as the source of suffering and limiting beliefs, as it creates the illusion of a separate self that is disconnected from the rest of the universe. While the ego can be a useful tool for navigating the physical world, it can also hinder our spiritual growth and prevent us from experiencing the world in its true form. Psychedelic substances have been used for thousands of years in spiritual practices to help individuals transcend their ego and connect with the divine. During a psychedelic experience, the boundaries between the self and the environment are dissolved, allowing individuals to experience a sense of oneness with everything around them. This can lead to profound insights about the nature of existence, as well as a deep sense of peace and interconnectedness. However, it is important to note that simply taking a psychedelic substance is not enough to transcend the ego. It requires a willingness to let go of limiting beliefs and surrender control to the experience. This can be difficult for many people, as it can feel like the loss of their sense of self. There are also risks associated with attempting to transcend the ego through psychedelic substances. It is important to approach the experience with reverence and respect, and to have a trusted guide or therapist present to help navigate any challenging experiences that may arise. Ultimately, transcending the ego requires ongoing spiritual practice and a commitment to personal growth. While psychedelic substances can be a powerful tool in this journey, they are not a shortcut or a guarantee of enlightenment. It is up to each individual to do the work of transcending the ego and living from a place of deep inner wisdom and connection to the world around them.

LIVING FROM THE SOUL

Living from the soul is a new way of life that is emerging from psychedelic experiences. It is a way of being that aligns with our true nature, rather than the limited identity created by the ego. When we live from the soul, we are in harmony with our deepest desires and the universe as a whole. In this subchapter, we will explore what it means to live from the soul and how we can cultivate this way of being in our everyday lives. Living from the soul means being fully present in the moment and connected to our innermost self. It involves letting go of past regrets and future worries, and instead, focusing on the beauty and meaning of the present moment. When we live from the soul, we are more tuned in to our intuition and inner wisdom, which can guide us towards our purpose and passions. One of the core aspects of living from the soul is aligning with our values and authenticity. We need to take the time to reflect on our beliefs and what resonates with us on a deep level. Rather than conforming to societal or familial expectations, we must seek to honor our unique paths and truths. Living from the soul requires radical self-acceptance, self-awareness, and self-compassion. Another important aspect of living from the soul is cultivating a sense of interconnectedness with all beings. When we recognize that we are all part of a larger whole, we can act with compassion and kindness towards others. This involves breaking down barriers of separation and judgment, and instead, embracing unity and empathy. Practices such as meditation, yoga, and mindfulness can help us live from the soul. These techniques help us cultivate present-moment awareness and connect with our inner selves. Psychedelic experiences can also provide insights and perspectives that can help us live from the soul. However, it's essential to remember that living from the soul is an ongoing process that takes time and effort to cultivate. In conclusion, living from the soul is a new way of being that is emerging from psychedelic experiences. It involves being present in the moment, aligning with our values and authenticity, and cultivating a sense of interconnectedness with all beings. By living from the soul, we can experience greater joy, purpose, and fulfillment in our lives.

IMPLICATIONS FOR SOCIETY AND CULTURE

The use of psychedelics for spiritual and therapeutic purposes has been gaining acceptance in Western society in recent years. As research continues to demonstrate the potential benefits of these substances, society and culture are slowly shifting towards a more accepting and open attitude towards their use. One of the implications of this shift is that more individuals are seeking out psychedelic therapy to treat a wide range of mental health conditions, such as depression, anxiety, and addiction. This is particularly significant as traditional forms of therapy are often inadequate in treating these conditions. With the right set and setting, psychedelic-assisted therapy can produce powerful healing experiences that can lead to lasting positive change. Another implication is that the use of psychedelic substances can lead to a sense of interconnectedness and empathy towards others, and this can help to transcend traditional social boundaries. This can lead to a more compassionate and understanding society that is more willing to work together and see each other as part of a greater whole. As society moves towards a more accepting stance on the use of psychedelics, legislation surrounding these substances is also beginning to shift. In recent years, several cities and states in the United States have decriminalized the possession and use of certain psychedelics, with more likely to follow in the coming years. It is important to note, however, that the use of psychedelics is not without risks, and individuals who choose to use them should take precautions to ensure their experiences are as positive as possible. Additionally, education surrounding safe use and the benefits of these substances should be prioritized in the process of societal and cultural acceptance. Overall, the implications for society and culture surrounding the use of psychedelics are significant and potentially transformative. As research continues to emerge, it is likely that the medical and spiritual benefits of these substances will continue to gain recognition and legitimacy.